Essential Oils for Winter

40 Warming Recipes for Diffusers

Table of Contents

Introduction

Our sense of smell is a very interesting ability. While our olfactory senses are nowhere near that of animals, it is still an amazingly powerful tool within the realm of human capabilities. It may surprise many to know that our sense of smell and our reaction to it is at its basest form, chemical.

Senses located in our nasal cavity detect the presence of chemicals in our environment and relays that information to the brain. When these vaporized chemicals reach our nostrils, they dissolve in the mucus lying just under the surface where specialized receptor cells detect and identify the odor and send the message to the limbic section of the brain.

While this is a rather oversimplified explanation of how our sense of smell works, understanding this fundamental element helps us to see why essential oils have had such a powerful impact on our physical, mental, and emotional state.

No one knows exactly when man discovered the significant value of essential oils play in enhancing our quality of life but using them has been a common practice in many civilizations for thousands of years. For the newcomer, the thought of using smells, scents, and odors for healing may seem a little far-fetched. However, over the years, science has proven that our olfactory systems carry a pretty powerful punch when it comes to our health and mental state.

Part of the reason for this is because the area of the brain responsible for identifying smells is in our limbic system; this same area is connected to our central nervous system and the very seat of our emotions, motivations, and even our memory. That's why you are often surprised that you can be walking down a street without a care in the world and suddenly get a whiff of something and can immediately be transported back to your childhood or some other powerful event in your past.

For this reason, essential oils have been a part of life for many millennia. From time memorial, they have been used in our cosmetics, our diets, and even in helping us to connect with our more spiritual being. So, it only stands to reason that they would be used to help keep us warm during those cold winter months.

Diffusing Essential Oils

There are many ways you can access the power of essential oils but probably the most common is through a method called aromatic diffusion. Diffusing is the process of distributing the molecules of the essential oils in the air where they can be inhaled and have a direct impact on the nerves sending signals directly to the brain. It is one of the fastest and safest ways of getting the best effects from essential oils.

Aromatic diffusion can be done in several ways. The easiest is through direct inhalation; simply open the bottle of oil and inhale. You can also place a drop or two of the oil in the palm of your hand, rub your hands together to warm the liquid, then cup your hands together over your mouth and nose and inhale deeply.

These methods help to promote a more positive mental and emotional state of mind. This is why we often find an inner sense of calm when we smell certain fragrances. How do you feel when you walk past a bakery and you catch the scent of freshly baked goods wafting through the air? Or how about the sensation you feel from the smell of a fresh orange? These scents help pave the way to a more balanced and sensually rewarding experience that can soothe you in many ways.

Keeping Warm With Essential Oils

As we continue to increase in our understanding of essential oils, more people have begun to realize their importance in helping us to have a more balanced lifestyle. We understand how they can enhance our physical wellness in a world where physical activity is limited, diets are not always the smartest, and toxins fill the air.

Essential oils also boost our spiritual awareness as well. Many do not realize that the common practice of burning incense only benefit us because of the essential oils infused into them. They have been a common practice in religious and spiritual ceremonies for countless generations as aids to transcend to a higher level of consciousness. These oils activate certain areas of the brain that connect us to our emotions on an even deeper level.

Many of these oils have been used in cleaning your home, and even in helping to enhance our beauty routines without ever being fully aware of what they were. How many times have you purchased home cleaners that have been infused with lemony freshness or the flowers of spring?

Read the list of ingredients on your favorite cosmetics and you'll find that fragrances are often included. It's not just putting the product on your skin that makes you feel good, it's also the scent of these oils triggering feelings in your brain as well.

There's no doubt that essential oils play a major role in all of these aspects of our lives but how is it, you might wonder, that these oils can be used to keep a body warm in the winter time?

There are some oils that literally feel warm on the skin. When using these oils, you must exercise caution as many have been known to cause a burning sensation if applied topically. A list of these oils can be found in Chapter four of this book. Other oils work by boosting the circulation of the blood.

When the blood flows freely throughout the body, you will naturally feel warm. Learning how to use these oils can keep you from having a cold and miserable season where all of your energy is spent trying to hibernate until the sun is in a position to bring you warmth once again.

Chapter 1 – What You Should Know About Essential Oils

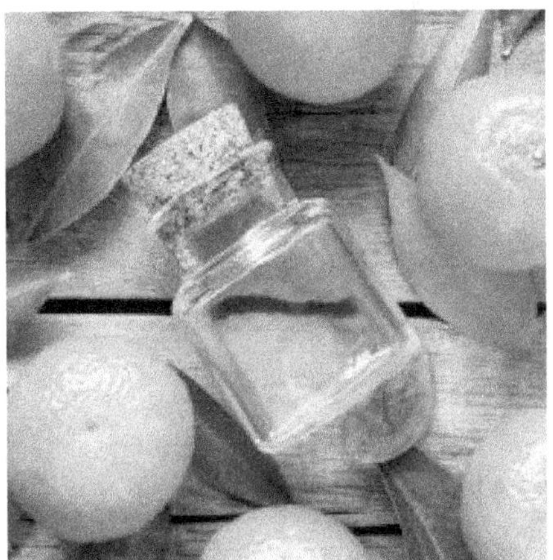

If you are new to the world of essential oils, it is important to first correct some commons misconceptions about them. First, and probably the most important thing to understand is that technically, essential oils are not considered to be real oils.

For a substance to be considered an "oil" it needs to be part fatty acid. It also needs to come from a plant that contains powerful medicinal and cosmetic qualities. So, while the fragrances coming from the plants in your garden may be appealing to your senses, if it doesn't have both medicinal properties and fatty acids it cannot be considered an essential oil.

That said, the majority of essential oils have been found to have many of the elements needed to fight off bacteria, fungus, and many viruses. So, the oils you learn are good for keeping you warm on those cold and chilly days are also very good in keeping your home clean and your air fresh.

It is also important to not confuse essential oils with fragrance oils. They are completely different. While essential oils come from our natural environment, fragrance oils are produced synthetically.

Even if you find on their ingredient list the term "natural" they are usually a synthetically derived compound designed to mimic those scents found in the natural environment. For the purposes of essential oils, they must be extracted from an actual plant. This helps us to understand why the cost of some essential oils can be so high.

It takes quite a few plants to produce even a small amount of essential oils. Depending on the oil you use, it could take as little as 100 pounds of plant matter to produce a single pound of essential oils.

Some oils require even more. For example, it can take as much as 4,000 pounds of Bulgarian roses to produce a single pound of its essential oil. This goes to show you that when you purchase your oils, you're purchasing a highly concentrated product than what you would normally be exposed to in nature.

This is also the reason why it is important that you exercise extreme caution when using these oils.

While they are usually recognized as safe, it is strongly recommended that they are combined with carrier oils like waxes, butters, or other natural forms of oil of dilution to cut their strength. When used at full strength, you could receive burns, rashes, and other unpleasant side effects. In any case, using these oils should be done sparingly for the best results.

Cautions

To that end, there are several precautionary warnings you need to keep in mind when using essential oils.

1. Oils like aniseed, rosemary, cedarwood, clary sage, cinnamon, clove, lemon, ginger, jasmine, nutmeg, chamomile, and sage should not be used if you or someone in your home is pregnant or nursing.

2. Always test your sensitivity to an essential oil before using it. You can do this by combining one drop of the oil in a ½ tsp. of olive, or jojoba oil and rubbing the solution on your upper arm. Let it remain there for a few hours checking regularly for the presence of a rash, redness, or itching. If after several hours, you have no reaction, it's likely that the oil is safe for you to use.

3. Treat any essential oils you have just as you would medications and keep them out of the reach of children. You also want to make sure that you avoid getting any of the oil in your eyes as it could cause damage.

4. While some of the essential oils listed are common ingredients in food recipes, never take the pure oil extract internally. Always remember that these are highly concentrated forms and can be extremely potent. Don't confuse the two. Those you buy in your local supermarket to use in food preparation have been well-diluted for safe use.

5. Don't overstock your oils. Most essential oils will last you up to five years (some only one or two) but keep in mind that when you use them you are only going to use a drop or two at a time. This means that if you purchase a large quantity of the oil in an effort to save money you may be throwing a good chunk of your investment away. Unless you know you're going to be using a large quantity of the oil throughout its lifespan, it is better to buy in smaller quantities so you get to take advantage of its full potency.

6. Finally, always do research before using any oil you're unfamiliar with. Keep on the lookout for allergies, and possible negative reactions for the first time you use it. There are over a hundred essential oils that are easy to obtain these days so if you're ever in doubt, avoid it completely. There are bound to be other oils that will give you the results you need without putting your health at risk.

Keeping these basic guidelines in mind and you'll be ready to start learning how to use essential oils during those harsh winter months to keep you warm.

Chapter 2 – How Essential Oils Warm the Body

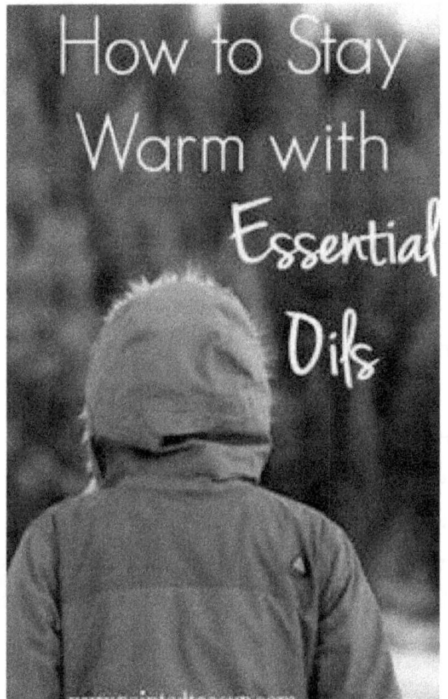

Wherever you live, when wintertime falls, it is difficult for many of us to focus on anything except getting warm. Whether you're fighting off extreme temperatures that dip below freezing or you're battling the unrelenting chill that silently creeps into every home during those frosty months the primary goal is to keep our bodies from tensing up when resisting the cold.

Some of us do this mentally, by slipping into a hibernation mode and burrowing ourselves under the covers where we can remain comfortable inside its warm folds. But for those, who have no choice but to rise and face the day no matter how much cold is on the ground, it is essential to find ways to keep warm in spite of the elements in our environment. It is for these people that the use of essential oils can prove to be invaluable.

These oils can stimulate your senses, uplift your mood, and increase the flow of blood running through your system; all of which can help to keep the body warm.

How They Fight the Chill

Often a person's sensitivity to cold has little to do with the changing climate but more to do with circulation. Many people who have a slow circulatory system will experience cold feet and hands, especially during the winter months. This is where essential oils can help. Certain oils can warm these extremities simply by applying one or two drops into a carrier oil, rubbing them into your cold hands and feet and you will immediately feel a warmth spread through your body.

While using these oils as a topical treatment can produce powerful effects, studies have shown that using them in diffusers can produce longer lasting results. In the next chapter, I'll discuss some of the many different ways you can diffuse essential oils but for now learning how they work is key.

How to Diffuse Essential Oils

One of the first things you'll hear when you're learning about essential oils is the term diffusion. This simply means of distributing the molecules of the oils into the air. This practice is an excellent way to get the maximum benefits out of these oils. There are several ways to diffuse essential oils; some may require you to purchase devices and other equipment while others do not. Let's talk about each one of these methods and what is needed.

Direct Inhalation

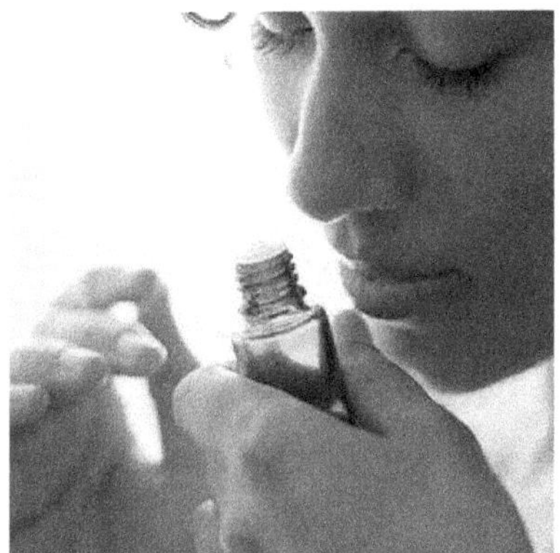

The key to successful diffusion is that the molecules of the oil permeate the air so they can be inhaled. There are at least three different ways you can diffuse through the air without a device.

1. If you have a small vial of the essential oil, the easiest way to get immediate effects is to place the open bottle up to your nose and then inhale deeply.

2. You can also place a few drops of the oil in the palm of your hand, rub your hands together vigorously, and then cup them together over your nose and mouth and inhale.

3. Place a few drops in a bowl of hot water or a hot bath and inhale the vapors.

Using a Cold Air Fan

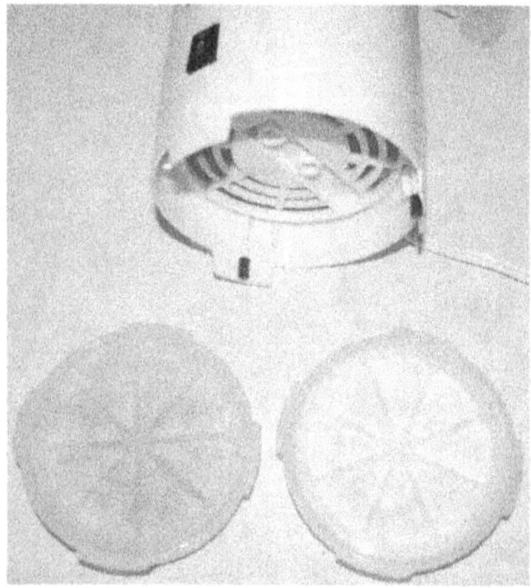

Cold Air fans are convenient and easy to use. The fan blows the cool air over a pad containing a few drops of the essential oil, which then releases the molecules into the air.

These fan diffusers come in a wide variety of sizes so you should be able to find one that will suit your specific needs. If you're planning to diffuse a small room then a small portable fan may be enough but if you need to diffuse a larger area, there are plenty to choose from.

The Ultrasonic Diffusers

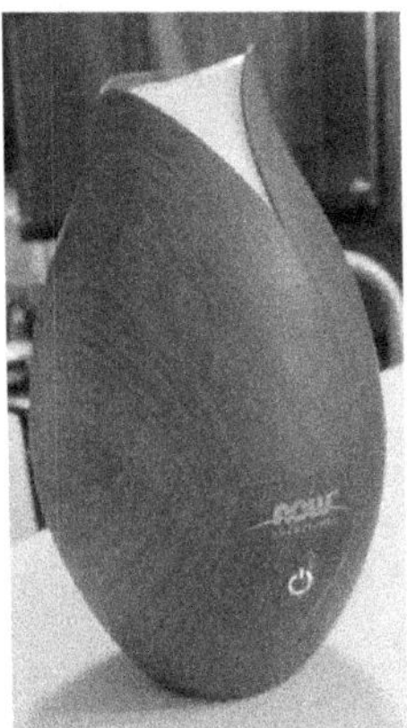

Ultrasonic diffusers are great when you want to combine the aromatherapy benefits of diffusing with the benefits of using a humidifier. You can thus, accomplish two health benefits with one device. These devices are capable of breaking up the essential oils into literally millions of tiny micro-particles and dispersing them throughout the air.

Atomizing Diffusers

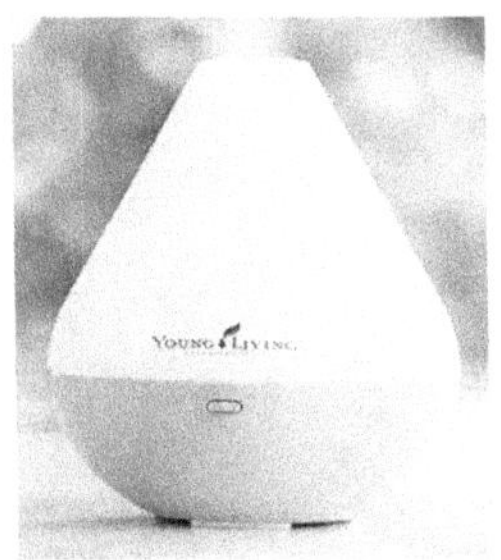

Atomizers have been around for centuries. They are popular because they don't need batteries or an electrical power source to work. Of course you can purchase all sorts of atomizers that can do everything from time the output of vapors throughout your day, have automatic shut offs, and a whole battery of additional features to get the job done but the most basic atomizer is simply a bottle with a spray component. Add the essential oil to the carrier oil and spritz in the air when needed.

Candle Diffusion

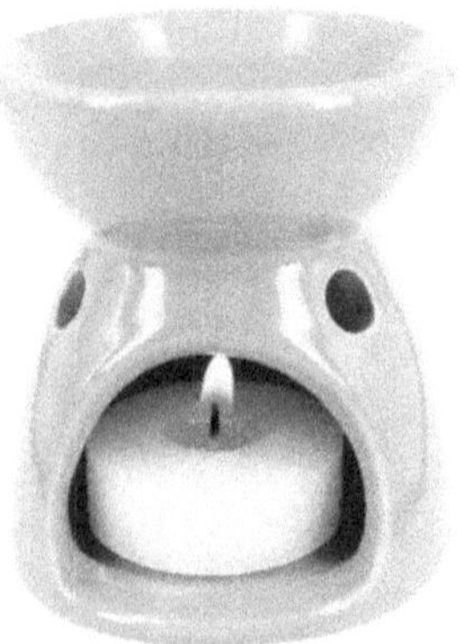

Candles can be an easy and pleasant way to diffuse essential oils. You can purchase candles already infused with the oils you want or you can make them yourself. Even plain unscented beeswax candles can work. Simply light a beeswax candle and let it burn for around five minutes. Blow out the candle and place a single drop of essential oil in the melted wax and relight.

Candle diffusion is easy and can be done anywhere it is safe to burn a candle. However, caution is warranted as essential oils are highly flammable.

Lamp Ring Diffusers

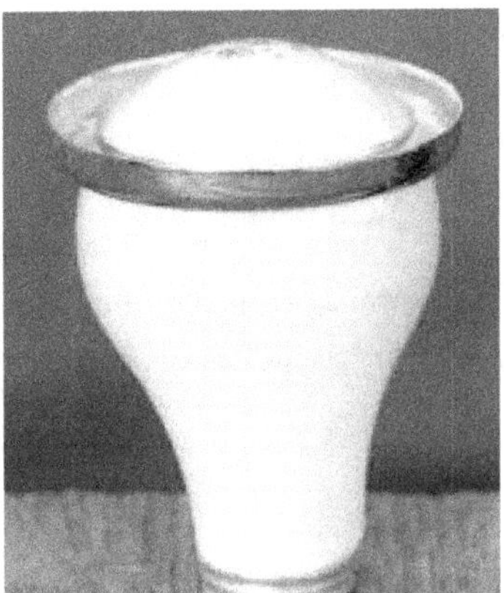

You can also find terracotta or brass lamp rings. These rings are designed to set directly onto a light bulb. They have a small lip where you can put a few drops of the essential oil. The heat from the bulb heats the oil and gently diffuses it into the air.

Diffusing essential oils is a tried and true method. If you are using diffusing devices of any type it is important that you follow the manufacturers directions carefully. While these are natural products, they are highly concentrated and flammable and could end up causing more harm than good if not used properly. Make sure that you use the right type of carrier oil or water solution for the device you use and you'll be able to get the most benefit from your aromatherapy.

Chapter 3 – The Art of Blending Essential Oils

We are all hard-wired to respond to certain aromas in the air. However, most of the aromas your olfactory lobe detects are not a single oil but instead a combination. To get the most out of your winter warming regime, you need to know how to blend your own essential oils to meet your specific needs.

Many of the oils listed at the end of this chapter have the ability to help with a lot more of the health challenges you face besides keeping you warm. Once you know how to mix and match, your essential oil treatments can provide you with a full battery of benefits.

There are several factors to keep in mind when blending essential oils. Once you understand these basic fundamentals you should be able to start mixing your own essential oils to personalize your results. Of course, this is only a basic guideline to get you started. For a more detailed study, there are a lot of books that you can refer to if you wish to pursue the practice further.

Fragrance Perception

To begin with you need to understand your own unique sense of smell. Some people are very sensitive to certain smells while others are not. One of the first things you must consider is how your own nose responds to the smells in your environment.

When you are deciding which oils should go in your warming blend make sure to choose those oils that you love and appreciate. Test them out, one at a time to make sure you're not choosing something that will have a negative effect on your mind and will still give you a pleasant feeling.

The Aromatherapy Song

Fragrances come in three notes that are very similar to the notes in music. One essential oil can either be a top, middle, or base note in the scent range.

Top Note: is the first recognizable impression your nose will detect when the aroma hits you. Its scent is usually powerful but it doesn't last very long.

The Middle Note: is the second recognizable scent you can identify. Its scent will linger a little longer than your top note (one to two hours) and represents the very heart of the aroma.

The Base Note: the final part of the blend is the base scent that will become apparent much later than the first and middle notes. It's the glue that holds all the scents together. The strength of your base note can help you to determine how long the effects of your blend will last.

One of the most important things you can do is to select each oil based on these three parameters to get the best possible results.

Proper Steps to Blending

Ideally, you should begin your process with five possible oils for your blend. Here are a few things to keep in mind to make sure that your blending is a success.

Step 1: To choose the right scents ask yourself these three questions:

1.   Do I enjoy the zest of fruit or the aroma of any herbs and spices?
2.   Are there any flowers that I specifically enjoy?
3.   Do I prefer the scents of natural greens like freshly cut grass or pines?

These questions will help you to zero in on the types of essential oils that will give you the scents and aromas you will enjoy.

Step 2: Now it's time to do a smell test.

1. Start by dropping a single drop of oil on a scent testing strip (these can be purchased online for as little as 100 strips for $5.00)

2. Slowly move the strip in a circular motion as you draw it up towards your nose stopping when it is about a foot away.

3. Make note as to what distance you begin to detect the aroma.

4. Then make a quick inhalation followed by a few deep and slow inhalations.

5. Make note of which aromas you detect immediately and which ones come later.

Step 3: Describe the effects of the aroma on you. This could include your thoughts, feelings, emotions, and moods the aromas evoke.

Step 4: Be aware of the sensations in your body. How does the fragrance enter your body? Does it move quickly up your nose? Does it invade the space between your eyes? Or do you feel it in you chest?

Step 5: Try to separate the five scents into notes. You should have one base note, two middle notes, and two possible top notes but sometimes you will find you can get better results with only two or three oils rather than using all five.

The Formula

The formula you use to create your own winter warming blend is to create a perfect balance for your unique makeup. This is done by first considering the strength of the oils you have. If you have one scent that is very strong you don't want to blend it with a milder scent. It will overpower it and you'll lose its beneficial effects. When you have a stronger scent you'll need to increase the ratio of the weaker scent to balance it out.

This requires you to choose the right ratio to balance all of the different oils. A good rule of thumb is to start with a total of 100 drops. This will make it easier to determine the percentage of each oil to be used in your blend. The good news is that there is no precise combination to get the effects you want; it is your formula so it is whatever you make it. If it is not exactly as you imagined it, you can always make adjustments.

As you create your formula make careful note of each step you take, the number of drops you use and always do a scent test at each phase of the blend. Be creative and daring and let your senses be your guide.

There are several different categories of essential oils so it would help to know the differences.

Citrus Oils are those that come from citrus fruits and include lime, mandarin, orange, and bergamot.

Green Oils are those that come from plants like basil, Immortelle, Oakmoss, and Violet.

Herbal Oils include basil, black pepper, clove, rosemary, and thyme.

Minty Oils include peppermint, spearmint, and sage

Floral Oils come from flowers like lavender, rose, and ylang ylang.

Warm Oils consist of anise, cedarwood, ginger, and marjoram.

Fruity Oils include pine, chamomile, and juniper

Sultry Oils include Jasmine, Tuberose, and Boronia

Once you've come up with your perfect blend you're ready to put it to the test. Don't be discouraged if you don't get the best results the first time.

The secret to the best blends is in the practicing but don't throw them out if they don't give you the effects you want. Essential oils have a lot of uses and you'll find a place for your new blend somewhere in your home or life.

While there are hundreds of different essential oils known to help with warming you up during those cold winter months, here is a list of some to start with.

Common Essential Oils Known for Warming

1. Angelica

2. Anise

3. Basil

4. Bergamot

5. Benzoin

6. Western Red Cedar

7. Cardamom

8. Citronella

9. Citrus

10. Clary Sage

11. Coriander

12. Cumin

13. Cypress

14. Dill

15. Dorado Azul

16. Eucalyptus

17. Douglas Fir

18. Idaho Balsam Fir

19. White Fir

20. Fleabane

21. Frankincense

22. Sacred Frankincense

23. Geranium

24. Ginger

25. Goldenrod

26. Grapefruit

27. Helichrysum

28. Juniper

29. Laurus Noblis

30. Lavender

31. Lemon

32. Lime

33. Mandarin

34. Marjoram

35. Mountain Savory

36. Myrtle

37. Nutmeg

38. Orange

39. Palo Santo

40. Black Pepper

41. Peppermint

42. Pine

43. Ravintsara

44. Rosemary

45. Sage

46. Spanish Sage

47. Spearmint

48. Spruce

49. Tangarine

50. Tarragon

Chapter 4 – Recipes for Warming Blends

With hundreds of essential oils to choose from there are literally thousands of possible combinations. If you're not ready to try blending your own, or you just want to get more familiar with these oils before you start, here are a few recipes to get you started.

Sugar and Spice

3 drops of sweet orange

3 drops of bergamot

2 drops of clove

2 drops of cinnamon.

Winter Wonderland

3 drops of pine

3 drops of cedarwood

2 drops of orange

2 drops of nutmeg.

Immunity Booster

3 drops of eucalyptus

3 drops of lavender

2 drops of thyme

2 drops of pine.

The Mint

5 drops of spearmint

2 drops of lemon

1 drop of lavender

1 drop of eucalyptus

1 drop of cedarwood.

Warm Woods

2 drops of myrrh

2 drops of pine

2 drops of frankincense

2 drops of cedarwood.

The Winter Sleep

3 drops of lavender

3 drops of orange

1 drop of thieves

3 drops of cedarwood

Holiday Fun

3 drops of orange

2 drops of peppermint

3 drops of frankincense

Holiday Candy

3 drops of lavender

3 drops of orange

1 drop of thieves

3 drops of cedarwood

Winter Warm Up

2 drops of lavender

2 drops of rosemary

2 drops of eucalyptus

3 drops of peppermint

Winter's Gift

3 drops of orange

5 drops of frankincense

4 drops of myrrh

The Fireplace

3 drops of blue spruce

4 drops of cedarwood

4 drops of pine

Winter Wonderland

5 drops of orange

5 drops of spruce

3 drops of pine

Beat the Winter Blues

10 drops of orange

5 drops of cedarwood

1 drop of ylang ylang

Winter Holiday

5 drops of balsam fir

5 drops of black spruce

2 drops of cedarwood

1 drop of juniper

Fall Warm Up

2 drops of cedarwood

3 drops of bergamot

A Walk in the Woods

2 drops cypress

2 drops of bergamot

Spicy Evenings

2 drops of white fir

2 drops of sandalwood

4 drops of cypress

The Rain

1 drop of lavender

2 drops of bergamot

3 drops of clary sage

A Winter Boost

2 drops of wintergreen

4 drops of citrus

A Clear Day

1 drop of patchouli

1 drop of sandalwood

2 drops of citrus fresh

2 drops of ylang ylang

 A Good Night

1 drop of cedarwood

2 drops of vetiver

4 drops of lavender

The Christmas Gift

3 drops of orange

5 drops of frankincense

4 drops of myrrh

Winter Tea

3 drops of orange

1 drop of nutmeg

1 drop of cinnamon

1 drop of clove

1 drop of cardamom

Winter Forest

2 drops of white fir

2 drops of orange

2 drops of cinnamon

The Winter Blues

8 drops of orange

5 drops of cedarwood

1 drop of ylang ylang

Winter Dreams

3 drops of cinnamon

3 drops of geranium

3 drops of vetiver

Winter Trees

3 drops of blue Spruce

4 drops of pine

4 drops of cedarwood

Christmas

3 drops of balsam fir

1 drop of grapefruit

2 drops of frankincense

Candy Cane

3 drops of wintergreen

1 drop of cinnamon

Minty Surprise

5 drops of peppermint

2 drops of ylang ylang

Winter Energy

3 drops of thieves

2 drops of peppermint

Winter Race

3 drops of nutmeg

3 drops of coriander

3 drops of frankincense

Christmas Time

4 drops of pine

2 drops of cypress

2 drops of orange

1 drop of nutmeg

The Thankful Heart

1 drop of ginger

1 drop of cinnamon

2 drops of coriander

1 drop of clove

A Winter Treat

3 drops of wild orange

2 drops of frankincense

2 drops of cassia

A Fall Warm Up

2 drops of wild orange

1 drop of clove

1 drop of ginger

1 drop of frankincense

For a Crispy Day

3 drops of wild orange

3 drops of patchouli

1 drop of clove

A Spicy Orange

3 drops of wild orange

2 drops of ginger

1 drop of cinnamon

Apple Pie

2 drops of clove

2 drops of cinnamon

2 drops of ginger

The Warm Calm

1 drop of rosemary

1 drop of clove

1 drop of eucalyptus

1 drop of cinnamon

1 drop of orange

As you read through each of these recipes, you probably noticed a repeating of some essential oils. Oils like cinnamon, cloves, lemon, lavender, eucalyptus, and citrus are the most commonly used and most readily available.

However, there are many other essential oils that may create an even more pleasant aroma in your diffuser. If you can find them at an affordable price, feel free to use them and experiment with your own blends of winter warming relief. You may even invent something that you'll want to share with others who are fighting off those winter chills.

Conclusion

Whether your feelings of cold come after spending your time out in the elements or from a slow circulatory system, essential oils may be the most natural solution to your problem. Rather than fighting off the tendency to go into hibernation mode or the frustration of never feeling warm these oils are natures way of balancing the scales and keeping everything as it should be.

It may be a new venture into getting an understanding of these oils and how they work but we hope that from the pages of this book you will find enough motivation and knowledge to at least get you started on warmer winter days so you can get the most out of the fun and holiday spirit and warm your body as much as you have warmed your heart.

FREE Bonus Reminder

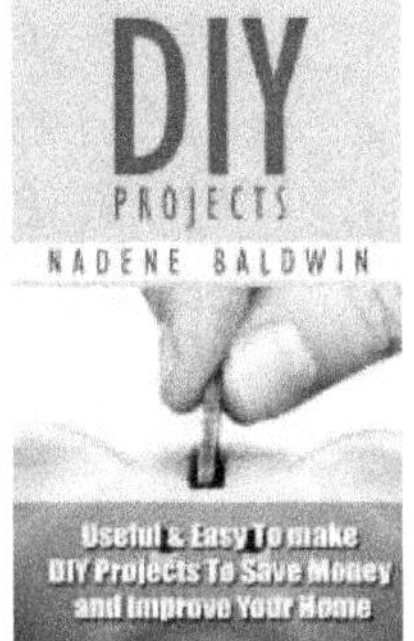

If you have not grabbed it yet, please go ahead and download your special bonus report *"DIY Projects. 13 Useful & Easy To Make DIY Projects To Save Money & Improve Your Home!"*

Simply Click the Button Below

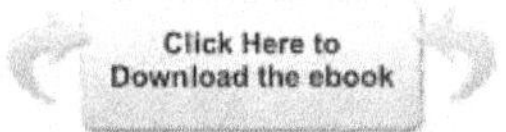

OR **Go to This Page**

http://diyhomecraft.com/free

BONUS #2: More Free & Discounted Books or Products

Do you want to receive more Free/Discounted Books or Products?

We have a mailing list where we send out our new Books or Products when they go free or with a discount on Amazon. Click on the link below to sign up for Free & Discount Book & Product Promotions.

=> Sign Up for Free & Discount Book & Product Promotions <=

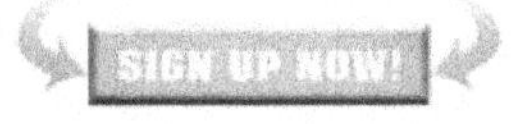

OR Go to this URL

http://zbit.ly/1WBb1Ek

www.ingramcontent.com/pod-product-compliance
Lightning Source LLC
Chambersburg PA
CBHW060822260726
48660CB00003B/1045